INTRODU

CW00796194

WEIGH

PSYCHOLOGY

FOR WOMEN

Kick the Fat Girl Out of Your Head and Lose Weight!

BY FELICIA URBAN RN, MSN

Published by

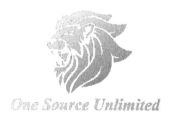

One Source Unlimited

Interested in more content by Felicia Urban?

Come visit us on the Weight Loss Psychology Series website and don't forget to hit that subscribe button to stay up to date on all new content!

https://WeightLossPsychologySeries.com

Interact with Weight Loss Psychology community by joining the Facebook page

https://www.facebook.com/WeightLossPsychologySeries

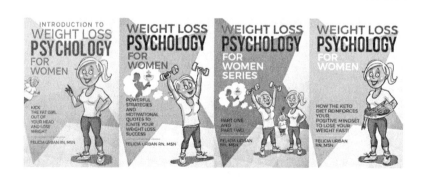

Felicia Urban RN, MSN

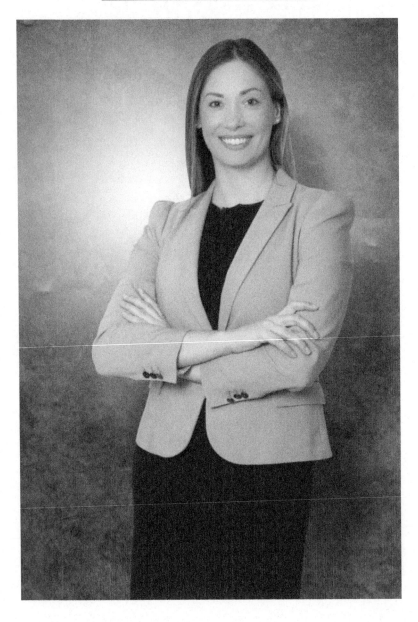

About the author

The author, Felicia Urban RN, MSN, suffered from weight loss and gain until she was thirty years old. At age 29, she was at her highest weight ever of 234 pounds.

She lost an amazing 90 pounds over the course of one year! She earnestly sought to understand what made her weight loss journey so difficult in the past and how to recapture and maintain her successful mindset that lead to her astounding 90-pound weight loss.

Her search led her to land a job at a popular weight loss physician's clinic. Here she interviewed and obtained the weight loss history of an estimated 500 plus patients who were all struggling to win the battle of permanent weight loss. One thing became clear to Ms. Urban, mindset prepping and maintenance of that mindset are essential to permanent weight loss success!

Most diets will work if followed closely. The difference between success and failure, Ms. Urban found, wasn't the diet plan, it was the proper mindset! Upon learning this, Ms. Urban has made it her life's mission to teach as many people as she can how to achieve proper mindset and reach their goals as she has done herself.

Ms. Urban lives on the outskirts of Orlando, Florida with her husband, three kids, four horses, three dogs and one cat named, "Frodo". She loves paintball, camping and growing organic vegetables. She now has a successful private practice as a weight-loss and life coach.

Introduction

Some diets allow you to eat anything you want, as long as you do so within a few hours in the day. Other diets allow you to eat cookies, but the truth is, those cookies taste like cardboard. There are so many tricks, hacks, and crazy regimens one can use to try and lose weight. The reality is, if the mindset is not there to lose weight, it is not going to happen.

Finding diets, learning about different foods, and understanding how weight loss occurs are all simple things that anyone can achieve. When it comes time to actually start losing the weight, however, that is when a lot of people drop out. The reason why so many people fail to keep up with their diets is not because of what foods they are choosing to eat or which spin class they are enrolled in. It is because their minds have not caught up to what their hearts actually want.

There is a root issue for why someone can't lose weight. Food for some people becomes a comfort that not everyone is ready to let go of. Whether someone hates eating veggies and only eats junk, or if someone binges healthy food, there is a reason why we all have our certain eating habits. By digging deep into our past, present, and goals for the future, we can discover that the key to losing weight is not in a pill or program. It is all in our head.

The Tools Needed

If you walk into any given store at any point the week after New Year's Day, there will likely be displays and areas filled with weight-loss gear, workout clothes, and everything you need to lose weight. There is this illusion that if you buy a bunch of workout stuff, the motivation to actually workout will follow. This method can work for some people, but for the most part, there are not exact tools needed to lose weight. You might use resistance bands, weighted ankle straps, and the cutest matching sports bra and leggings set, but the weight is not going to come off unless you have reached the right mindset.

The only tool necessary to lose weight is your brain. You can find ways to work out without any gear or extra supplements. These certainly help make things easier, and many people find help from having different tools of motivation. The key—the most important tool of all—is a mindset that is ready to confront the issues and work through them in order to achieve weight-loss goals.

Having a clear goal as well as a plan of attack are the next two important tools needed to make sure that you are going to be able to lose the weight once and for all, as well as the tools needed to make sure the weight does not come back.

Take Your Time

Weight loss is a journey, not just a weekend trip. That being said, it is going to take some time to actually achieve your goals. You likely won't find it to be an easy, casual journey either. You are going to run into some bumps and slipups that might make it hard to recover. There are going to be moments when you ask if it is worth it all in the end and other times where you question why you are even doing what you are. It is not going to be an easy or quick thing. If it were, you would have done it by now.

All of this is important to accept when beginning a weight-loss regimen. Accept the fact that there is no small fix for weight loss. There are pills you can take that help a bit, and other supplements that might help you lose some pounds. To really change your life and finally become the person you have always wanted to be, however, it is going to take some time. Weight loss is a process that requires patience, acceptance, and dedication. Though it might be tough at first, it does get easier. Achieving your goals is ALWAYS worth it in the end.

Table of Contents

<u>Chapter 1 – Looking Inward</u>

Sometimes, our weight-loss goals are all about just making sure that we look good in a bikini. Though we want our outsides to look good, we have to make sure the insides are looking even better. This does not mean your bones and blood, but your heart and mind. Is your brain ready to go through such a journey? Is your heart really in it in the end?

If you want to make sure you look good, you can't expect to do so while completely disregarding the inner workings of all the other systems in your body. This journey should be a healthy one, and that does not mean just looking the part. Crash dieting, binging and purging, and using extreme weight-loss supplements are all just attempts at fixing something that weight loss will not cure.

What's more important than just making sure you can fit into the right-sized outfit for an upcoming wedding is making sure that your mental state is strong enough to handle it if you don't end up fitting. The first step in doing this is making sure that you look at the root issue rather than looking at what you see in the mirror.

Identifying Trauma

Losing weight means looking at our past lives to determine what might have caused our current bad behaviors. Sometimes, this means having to look at a specific childhood trauma. Trauma can be defined as any sort of disturbing, unsettling, or distressing occurrence. Sometimes, this one small instance sticks with us forever, such as a car accident or natural disaster. Other times, trauma presents itself in other forms such as having an abusive or alcoholic parent.

You might already realize your traumas, or maybe it will take some time to understand the things you endured as a child that still disturb you as an adult. In order to make sure that you can combat everything that might come your way as you work out, it is important to determine what trauma still follows you. Perhaps you eat when you feel stressed because, as a child, you would eat snacks in the kitchen while your parents fought in the other room. Maybe you can't go to the gym because it is located next to a dentist's office, and you had a traumatic teeth-cleaning experience as a child. Knowingly or not, your trauma is likely playing into your current eating and dieting habits.

Confront the Root Issue

The thing about most of our problems is that you can usually trace them back to one big issue. We're like trees. We have all these branches, leaves, and little inner workings that all lead back to the trunk. Without that big deep root, nothing else would exist. For the most part, we can trace our current issues back to one, or maybe two root issues.

For example, many control issues come from a place of fear of abandonment. Those that look for ways to take control of their lives, whether it is in work or social settings, usually can trace their issues back to a time when they felt like they had no control. Maybe a parent left, or they dealt with loss at a young age. This control might come into play in their eating habits as well. By identifying past traumas and looking inward, you will be surprised at how easily you can confront the root issue to most of your problems.

This is not always going to be the case with everything in life. Certain illnesses or money issues are things that might spring up later in life, and we can't always connect these issues to our childhoods. When it comes to eating, however, that is usually an emotional experience for someone, which means they can trace it to their past life and analyze how or why that specific eating habit was created.

Why do I Eat?

Before dieting, continue with your current eating habits. Take note while you are eating about how it makes you feel. If you are sitting on the couch and you decide to eat the entire bag of chips when it only takes a handful to feel full, make a note of why you decided to do that. You won't always be able to attack the root issue right away, but you might start determining why you feel the need to overeat when you know you shouldn't. Maybe you will realize you are only eating because you are bored, or perhaps it is just a habit of convenience. Maybe you realize that you don't even feel that good while eating the chips, but you do it anyway.

Always ask why whenever you are eating. Why am I choosing to eat this fast food when there is food in the fridge? Why am I eating two sandwiches when it only takes one? Why do I keep eating this dip even though I'm already full? The more you ask why and question the behaviors you are able to identify, the better you will be able to come up with a solution to confront and attack your root issues.

Finding a New Goal

What's your goal for losing weight? Is it to fit into a dress? Is it so you can get a new boyfriend/girlfriend? Is it so you have a flat stomach or so your face is not as round? If your goal for losing weight is just to look good, you should find a new goal. That is the reason many people want to lose weight in the first place. They just want to be "hot" or "sexy," with a fit body that attracts other people, or at least gets positive attention from those around them. It is not uncommon to have vanity goals when it comes to losing weight. It is also not uncommon for people to give up on their weight-loss goals.

Looking good should just be an added bonus for losing weight. If you don't find a substantial and deeply-rooted goal for losing weight, you won't be as likely to keep up with your hopes. Instead of losing weight just to be hot, you have to find a reason that is more important.

Lose weight because you want to have a healthy heart. Having a healthy heart means that you will live longer, which means you'll get to spend more time with your friends and family. When you create a goal that has more meaning, you will be able to stick to that goal more easily than if you just want to be able to slip into some skinny jeans.

Create smaller goals that are important as well. Lose the weight because you want to be able to walk up a flight of stairs without having to catch your breath. Lose weight because you want to make it easier to move when it comes time to switch apartments. Lose weight because you will have the assurance that you can outrun anyone in case of some sort of zombie apocalypse.

Just remember that looking the best out of everyone at your high school reunion will just be the added bonus to losing weight, not the overall goal. That way, you will be able to stick to your weight-loss regimen if you do hit a certain body weight.

It is also important to understand your current value and beauty. You are not ugly, unattractive, or undesirable at any weight. That beautiful person exists inside of you, and it will show through no matter what size you are. You just have to recognize that wonderful person and treat them well, not shame them for not looking "sexy" enough.

Other Benefits

When creating a goal, you have to look at the overall benefits that will come along with achieving certain milestones. By doing this, you will be able to fulfill your goals better because you have a clear map of what benefits you will be reaping.

There are so many benefits to losing weight besides just the way you might look. Losing weight could help someone manage with their anxiety and depression. Working out releases endorphins, and certain junk food has been linked to producing depressive feelings.

Being more in shape allows someone to do things that someone out of shape, can't. You can go for walks with friends and not have to worry about what games you might play that could involve physical activity.

Being an overweight teenager and young adult is challenging because, at that age, there is so much pressure to look good. However, being overweight and in your forties or older is so much worse, and not even for beauty reasons. As our bodies age, no matter how healthy they are, certain things just don't work the way they used to. Our backs, knees, and hips start to not work as well as they used to and being overweight just puts more pressure on all these parts of our bodies. The older you get, the harder being overweight is on your body. It is also harder to lose weight the older you get. Losing the weight now, no matter what age, is always a better option than waiting and losing the weight later.

Avoid Triggers

Once you start identifying your trauma, it is time to look at what triggers might cause you to keep slipping up on your goals. This might include a bakery that you have to pass on your way home from work. Maybe different parties you frequent have buffet-style snacks always readily available. When you can start to identify what triggers surround you that cause you to eat, you can do your best to avoid these triggers, or at least be ready when they come about.

This might also include certain behaviors, experiences, or even people that make you feel like you have to eat. Maybe whenever you get in a fight with your boyfriend/girlfriend, you cope by binging out on some ice cream. Perhaps you feel like you can't sit down to watch a movie without having a snack in your hand. There are many different triggers we have on an individual level, but the main idea is that they need to be identified so it is easier to either avoid or confront them.

Avoiding Punishment

The biggest mistake we make when starting any sort of diet or weight-loss regimen is that we punish ourselves along the way. Whether the punishment comes from us not starting at the right time, slipping up on a strict diet, or just being regretful for not starting sooner, most of us are way too hard on ourselves. We say things to ourselves that are crueler than our worst bullies could imagine.

When we punish ourselves, whether it is just saying mean things in our heads or actually self-harming, we're forcing ourselves to feel dangerous emotions that might cause us to eat. Maybe you are mad at yourself for eating the free donuts your coworker brought into work. As a punishment that day, you skip lunch. On a more extreme level, maybe you hate yourself so much for being overweight for a long time that you go as far as to physically self-harm yourself.

Punishment is necessary for training dogs or teaching kids certain lessons. We punish bullies, criminals, and other people that exhibit bad behavior. You don't need to punish yourself, however. You should be your own best friend, so instead of making yourself feel terrible for not reaching a goal, remind yourself that you need to take care of yourself because you deserve it.

We still have to stay strict with our goals, but positive reinforcement will always be better than tearing yourself apart. When you constantly belittle yourself, you are seeing yourself as someone that does not deserve happiness. You might be so hard on yourself that you get to a point where you question whether you even deserve to have a healthy body.

Go at your own pace and start dieting and exercising when you are ready. Right now, however, you have to make a promise to yourself that you are going to go a little easier on yourself. No more calling yourself dumb, lazy, or ugly. When you look in the mirror, remember to point out the things you like, reminding yourself of how much beauty you really do have to offer. It is an uncomfortable feeling for some, but it is incredibly important in order to make sure that you fulfill your weight-loss goals.

Small Wins and Losses

Having an overall goal is important, but make sure to set small goals in between. For example, maybe your overall goal is to lose fifty pounds in a year. A small goal, then, would be to lose five pounds. Instead of waiting to celebrate until you lose the big fifty, have five- or ten-pound milestones. Celebrate that you are doing it! Just knowing you need to start living healthier is a huge thing, as not many people are willing to admit to themselves that they need to lose some weight and eat healthier. Once you actually start doing it, that is even more amazing! You should be incredibly proud, and the continual encouragement will only help you achieve your goals much easier in the end.

If you do slip up and do something that goes against your diet and exercise plan, just look at it as a small loss and not a complete failure. By reminding ourselves that we just made a small mistake, we can find the courage to keep going. When we tell ourselves we failed and have to start over, it can be hard to get back on track. Accept that you are going to have small losses along the way and remember that you will have just as many small victories.

Positive Reinforcement

Some instances require tough love, but that is not always going to work when it comes to losing weight. There are some people that are really hard on themselves, and it works to stick to a diet and exercise plan, but they might not be happy overall. The way to actually have a healthy body and a happy mind is to use positive reinforcement on yourself.

We get enough heat from the world we live in as it is. Our parents might be a source of "tough love," or maybe it is just the way that society makes some of us feel. We get enough of a feeling that we might not be "good enough" from other sources such that we don't need to do that to ourselves either. The key to having a consistent weight-loss mindset, geared towards achieving goals, is to use positive reinforcement.

Chapter 2 - Recent Mindset Research

Doing research is an important part of a weight-loss journey. Certain things might pose a health risk. If you try crash dieting, starvation periods, or other dangerous supplements, you might run the risk of doing more harm than good to your body. Before starting a serious weight-loss plan, it is always important to consult a physician. What might work for one person could be a dangerous risk for another. No two bodies are alike, so we can't always make assumptions about effects or results for different people participating in a weight-loss regimen.

What's more important is doing research on one's brain. Sometimes, that can be overlooked. When we lose weight, or at least when we start thinking of how we're going to cut the fat, we look at our stomachs and muscles, hoping to reduce the size of every physical element of our body. What's more important than improving on our muscles and other parts of our bodies is making sure that we're improving what's going on in our mind as well. It is easy to see that the way that we see food and ourselves is dependent on how our brain works. It goes much deeper than that, however.

There is an emphasis on mindset research, as it is clear that there is not yet a trick to losing weight. Instead of looking at how certain foods might affect our different body parts, we need to start looking at how food affects our mind. In addition to that, we need to look at our behavior, the choices we make, and the ways that we perceive different people and events in order to determine what the problem might be in our weight-loss journey. This emphasis also helps us to discover new ways to lose weight. It is not an answer of what our calorie count is, or how many minutes we clock at the gym. The key to achieving all of our weight-loss goals is hidden inside our brain, and scientists know this.

Being aware of the science behind a weight-loss mindset can help an individual be sure that they will actually find success with their plan. If we continue to ignore our brains and instead just workout our arms, abs, and legs, we'll never find easy success. It will always be about forcing ourselves to go to the gym, or moments of binging followed by punishment purging. By changing our mindset and the way we see food, as well as our perceptions of ourselves, we can make it easy to actually stick to a plan that helps us shed pounds and keep them off forever.

You Are Not Alone

Weight loss can be a lonely journey. It is up to us to get started, and we can only rely on ourselves to make sure that we follow through. It is likely that moments of loneliness are what led to our weight-loss struggles in the first place. Having to depend on just ourselves in this struggle can be what keeps us from achieving our goals. Sometimes, we are not strong enough to handle it all on our own, and that is okay. We need to remember that at first, we might need to ask for help. We shouldn't be expected to do it all by ourselves. When we become too dependent on ourselves for things that we can't always fix alone, there is a feeling of shame when we can't follow through.

When going through this journey, always remember that you are not alone. More than two in three adults are considered overweight. At this point, more people are struggling with their weight than those that are not. Even people that are not overweight still struggle with their perception of themselves as well as their overall body image. Don't be afraid to reach out and ask for help. Find a friend that also might be struggling with their weight and see if they want to start going on walks with you. The Statistics prove that we are not in this alone, so there is no shame in reaching out for help.

One in thirteen adults have extreme obesity. When looking at weight-loss statistics like that, it is clear to see that you are certainly not alone in your weight-loss struggles. While these numbers might be concerning for our overall health and the way in which our society evaluates us, it can also be comforting to know that there are plenty people around us going through the same struggle. It is also a reminder that it is not our fault we got this way. We're certainly complicit in our own choices and can't blame the world for all of our health issues. It is a comforting reminder, however, to know that we're in a world set up for our weight issues. When a fast food meal is cheaper than a salad, we can't be so hard on ourselves when we do have moments of weakness.

How Being Overweight Affects Your Mind

Anyone can have a fit body, but that doesn't always mean they have a healthy mind. Mental illness like bipolar disorder, depression, and anxiety have the ability to affect many different people, no matter their size. With that in mind, it is also important to know that being overweight can have some seriously negative effects on your brain. Someone that struggles with mental illness and who is overweight might find that shedding some pounds actually improves their overall mental health as well.

Those who are overweight have issues with depression and anxiety more often than physically fit individuals. Part of this is because of the way society treats overweight individuals. When thin models are plastered all over billboards and other advertisements, it can be hard to not have a warped perception of bodies that don't look the same as those airbrushed beauties. However, more so than just the way our society affects body image, there are physical effects being overweight has on the brain.

Being overweight might lead to a higher risk of getting Alzheimer's or dementia. This is partially because excess weight affects the hippocampus, which we'll discuss in the next section. The foods that we eat, and how much oxygen we're giving our body, increase and decrease certain chemical levels in our brain which, in turn, may cause mental illnesses and disorders. These can end up leading to more weight loss on top of that as well.

There is a "dulling" effect on those who are overweight which leads to less enjoyment and pleasure from eating certain foods. When we drink sugary drinks all day, we become used to that constant sugar intake. This ends up warping our perception on sugary sweets, which means we get used to them and end up wanting more. In order to understand how this dulling effect works, start by giving up just one food you eat all the time. Before you start with a full-on diet, just give up something "bad for you" that you eat a few times a week. After just a week free of your item of choice, go ahead and indulge. You will be shocked at how sweet it might taste. This is because you have reduced your tolerance. The pleasure from just that one drink is so much greater than the consistent level of gratification you get from giving into your frequent indulgence.

The striatum is a part of our brain that is responsible for pleasure regulation. In overweight individuals, especially women, the striatum becomes weakened, giving us less pleasurable responses. This means that in terms of more than just food, we'll receive less pleasure from things that normally would bring us great joy. By eating healthier and exercising regularly, we're also taking care of our striatum which means our pleasure levels will rise back to where they should be. This is pleasure in all forms, whether it is from food, family, friends, music, sex, or anything else that brings us joy and happiness. The healthier our striatum, the more pleasure we'll feel.

The Effects on the Hippocampus

The hippocampus can actually grow with exercise. This part of your brain is responsible for the regulation of emotions. Those who struggle with their weight likely have some issues controlling their emotions, which will usually end up leading to more unhealthy eating patterns. When our emotions are out of whack, we make decisions we would not normally make with a clear head. This is when diets can really get messed up and lead to more weight gain and disappointment.

Those who are overweight have been known to have a lower ability to remember things, especially those aged eighteen to thirty-five. When our memory is warped, it can lead to plenty of other serious issues. We might forget how much we ate in a day, meaning we're not regulating our intake. We could also forget that we have not eaten, which is also a very unhealthy eating pattern. When we don't track how much we've been eating, it can end up causing cravings that can lead to sneaky weight gain.

Memory performance has been shown to improve in those that lose weight. Memory plays a role in weight management, as sometimes, our perspective on when to eat and when we last ate can be pretty hard to keep up with.

Post-traumatic stress and depression can cause damage to the hippocampus. Those that experience these mental illnesses, as well as individuals that are overweight, will only hurt their brain more, causing other dietary issues to arise. Our brains are precious organs that should be cared for meticulously. Luckily, our hippocampus can be improved if we work it out!

This is done through healthy diets that provide the brain with the nutrients it needs to function. Exercise is also an important part of working out your brain. Doing brain exercises, such as mindfulness strategies or games like Sudoku or word searches, will also improve cognitive function that will lead to other important health benefits other than just a reduction in weight.

Sneaky Addictive Foods

Losing weight sometimes has to be treated like an addiction. Those who are dependent on drugs, alcohol, sex, or other addictive substances share some qualities with individuals that might also be addicted to food. Someone that is addicted to alcohol first has to quit drinking, and then they can work on their mental health in order to make sure that they are keeping up with their sobriety. A person that is addicted to food can't just quit eating! There will always be temptations for an alcoholic in social settings, bars, and even the liquor section at grocery stores. Food is so much more present, however, and we have to eat it every single day of our lives, multiple times a day, in order to continue living!

The key to kicking a food addiction is to cut out the foods that you are addicted to. The habit of eating is an addiction in itself, and that is something different that needs to be confronted. However, there are certain foods that are physically addictive that can be very challenging for a person to give up. Avoiding these addictive foods is the key.

The most addictive foods are filled with refined carbohydrates and added fat and sugar. This is because when those foods are eaten, there is a big increase of blood sugar which signals the pleasure centers of your brain, making you want even more. The reason why fast food is so good is because it is completely loaded with sugar. Even though Whoppers and Big Macs are not considered sweets, they still have a ton of added sugar that makes these foods addictive.

14

Tackling addiction is up to the individual. Some people are fine if they practice moderation. Other people can't even look at the food that they consider their addiction. In order to ensure that you don't fall back into a food addiction, it is important to figure out your plan for recovery. Are you going to be able to continue to surround yourself with the foods that tempt you on a daily basis? Or will you need to completely cut cupcakes out of your life? Sometimes, confronting addiction might also mean seeking professional help. There are psychologists that specialize in eating disorders who can provide extensive help to individuals with food addictions. There are also support groups filled with people that find themselves to be dependent upon or addicted to different foods and eating habits.

Chips and crackers are incredibly addicting for many reasons. They have added salt, which our bodies love, and they are not that filling on their own, meaning you will just keep loading up on them. Snacking is important to keep up our metabolism, but it needs to be extensively evaluated by the individual that is doing the snacking. Is it being done because you are actually hungry, or are you just bored? Maybe you are feeling anxious and need something to fill your hands, or perhaps you just looked at the snack and decided that it looked good.

Sweets like cake and ice cream are dangerous because of all the fat and sugar. If you are seriously addicted to sugar, you might also endure withdrawal symptoms when you don't get enough. Grumpiness, headaches, and other dangerous cravings are common symptoms of sugar addiction, so it is important that this individual issue is addressed in a weight-loss journey as well. You have to consider all of your dependencies and addictions in order to come up with a weight-loss plan that actually works.

How You Were Raised Counts

Those who have been overweight all their lives go through certain cycles. There is a period of unhealthy habits, the recognition that there needs to be a change, an attempt at change, the failure to follow through, and then back to a period of unhealthy habits. This cycle is present in many people that are overweight, but for those that were overweight kids and teens, it might be better understood. We might have also adopted this unhealthy cycle from our parents. Once we've found ourselves in this dangerous position, it can feel like clawing our way out when we actually decide we want to lose weight. If the pattern of behavior is not at first recognized, then we won't be able to determine the best method of breaking this unhealthy habit.

Studies have proven that kids who were weight-shamed go through cycles of binge eating and meal skipping that leads to self-loathing. A child that experiences criticism from their parents will start learning unhealthy methods of coping with weight and dieting. Eating is something that we've been doing all our lives, so the way that we eat now is certainly related to the way that we used to be taught to eat. Parents that might have body-shamed their kids by telling them they needed to lose weight or stop eating so much are responsible for causing self-loathing later in life.

Weight-shaming is not just blatantly telling someone that they are fat. It might also cloud diet encouragement. If your mom or dad always told you to try out a diet or suggested that you shouldn't eat a certain food, that was probably enough for you to feel a certain amount of shame about your weight. Even having a parent that continually talks about dieting is likely to make a child feel as though they should diet, too.

Many kids might grow up with moms who are constantly trying out new diets and fads. By seeing this is a kid, we end up going through the same phases. Maybe a parent was always saying things like, "I need to start my diet on Monday." This idea gets it in the kid's head that diets are something they should aim for, but only at a moment of convenience. The way a parent or even older sibling always talked about their body will play into how you might see your own body now. Perhaps your mom was always saying things like, "I hate my thighs; they are so big!" If a girl looks in the mirror and sees she has the same- shaped thighs as her mother, she'll end up thinking about how both she and her mother see those thighs as big, even though the mother never said anything directly to the girl about her body.

It is challenging because most parents just think they are helping. Parents that stock the fridge with Diet Coke instead of regular might think they are doing everyone a favor, when really, they are still supplying a form of addiction. Those that make sure to weigh their kids or track their workout routines could be doing so just because they want to make sure their kid is healthy, but they might not realize they are actually setting them up in a fearful manner in which dieting and exercising are an authoritative issue. Parents who are strict with routines might raise kids that don't have any routine at all as an act of rebellion.

How our parents diet, exercise, and talk about health in general will also form our own body perceptions. A daughter of a mother who consistently crash diets and works out too hard will likely produce a daughter that does the same. A father that only eats microwave meals or fast food is setting his kids up for doing the same when they become adults. When this happens, it is an insidious issue that we might not even recognize. The things our parents do can seem normal to us, as it is behavior that we learn is standard.

17

Be mindful of how you talk about exercise around children. Whether they are your kids or someone else's, never talk about body issues around kids. If you walk around talking about how much you hate your belly flab, you are teaching the kids around you to evaluate their own stomachs, wondering if they, too, have too much belly flab. Kids will be confronted with these body issues in other ways, as it is inevitable. As parents, caretakers, or any sort of role models, we should be teaching our kids how to love their bodies and properly take care of them because they deserve to be healthy, not because they should be skinnier or prettier.

Pregnant Moms Who Exercise Will Likely Give Birth to Healthy Kids

A study was conducted in which one group of pregnant rats were given exercise wheels, while another group of pregnant rats wasn't given anything. Those who used the exercise wheels ended up giving birth to more active babies. The babies of the moms that didn't work out would sit around and not do anything, as opposed to the babies of the moms that were always using an exercise wheel, who would use the wheel themselves. This was true for at least half of the rats born from active mothers. They weren't given anything else, so there weren't any factors to determine the difference in the level of activity other than the environment in which they were raised in the womb.

This exercise was inspired from similar research done on humans, though many scientists wonder if the effects were just because of a mother's influence after birth. Instead of assuming that it was from the active pregnancy, many scientists speculate that the difference in the amount of desire for physical activity is because mothers with active pregnancies are also mothers with active lives. It is clear that their lifestyle and habits can affect children, but the study with the rats proves that it might be on a level different than just the learned behavior.

Even in the womb, our mothers are teaching us how to exercise. We learn before we're even walking how important exercise is in maintaining a high level of physical activity. If a mother is more active while she's pregnant, she's setting her unborn baby up for a future in which it is just generally more active. This means that not only are we affected by the learned habits of our parents, but how we are actually created and grown also determines how much physical activity we let into our life.

Look back on your mother, father, or any other person that helped raise you, biologically or not. Were they active? Did they let that level of activity negatively affect your life? Did they reject exercise and healthy eating at all costs? Did you learn your unhealthy eating habits, or are they just a product of not being taught anything at all? We are taught how to eat and exercise, which means we are also taught *how not* to eat healthy or exercise. We can't fully blame our parents for the way we live now, but it is still important to recognize as it'll help bring us closer to closure with the unhealthy person in our head.

This is good motivation for any woman hoping to get pregnant in the future. Starting a family is a goal for many different people. An important aspect in starting that family is making sure to have a high level of physical activity. Kids require a lot of chasing and lifting. It is much harder for those that are not in shape to look after and give proper attention to active kids. It is also important to be healthy when pregnant with them in order to get them started right away with a healthy lifestyle. After kids are born, parents are also responsible for making sure their kids understand how to live a healthy lifestyle that does not include any bad habits.

Mindfulness Training Helps

Extensive research is being done on the positive effects of mindfulness and meditation. When a person is conscious of their surroundings and what their eating habits might be, they are more aware of the factors that make up for the fundamentals of why they are eating. Mindfulness is an attempt at a person putting emphasis on their surroundings and what's physically happening at any given time. Mindfulness is all about not thinking of the future or ruminating about the past. Reminiscing and planning are not harmful, but doing too much of either thing can certainly be.

Maintaining a diet can be the biggest problem for those who embark on a weight-loss journey. When a person is mindful, they will better be able to control their current situation instead of worrying so much about the past or future. When a person is mindful, they can better control their own thoughts and emotions rather than feeling overwhelmed by all their thoughts. If someone is always anxious about the future, they are going to be very worried about keeping up with their diet. They are taking on feelings of future failure instead of focusing on how to actually prevent that failure in the present moment. When we're not mindful, it can lead to moments of stress and anxiety that will lead to overeating or punishment purging.

The biggest way to be mindful about eating is to not do it while you are doing something else. Instead of sitting down in front of the TV, try to eat at a table where you can talk to someone else. If you focus on the show rather than how much you are eating, you are likely to continually stuff yourself until you are in pain rather than carefully tracking how much you are eating. You might grab a bag of chips when a movie starts, and before you know it, you are only halfway through the movie but all the way through the bag. The best way to be mindful when you eat is to just focus on only eating. This can be more enjoyable when meals are shared as well.

Appreciate the food that you are eating. In order to practice mindful eating, take in every bite slowly and focus on how it makes you feel overall rather than on what you might be doing later. Taste the food and savor each bite. Think of the work that went into creating that meal and the positive effects the food is going to have on your body. When we put an emphasis on this rather than on other things, we eat much slower which means we end up digesting better.

Sometimes, we eat so fast that we still feel hungry, so we end up going back for more. Instead, eat slowly so that you can feel yourself getting full rather than just trying to eat as much as possible. Take a break in between portions in order to ensure you are not just eating because you can. If you eat a lot of food in a quick amount of time, you are just setting yourself up for a night of misery.

Not only does this help someone in their weight-loss journey, but it can have very positive effects on other areas of one's life as well. Being mindful is not important just to shed pounds. It is also crucial to making sure you are actually living in the moment and enjoying your surroundings. Sometimes, eating might be a way to distract ourselves from different forms of pain. If we're mindful of that pain and how to overcome it, we're not only better off in our life in general, but we also eliminate the urge to eat when we aren't hungry.

Portion Control

Some restaurants use large portion sizes to give the illusion that they are giving you more for their money. Fast food restaurants, as well as sit-down chains, will advertise huge portions, boasting about burgers that are a quarter of a pound. This kind of "more for your money" mentality is present in all forms of capitalism, but it is dangerous when it is in terms of food. The larger the drink you get at the movies, the more money you save. Why get a medium when a large is only a quarter more? We think we're getting such a great deal for our money, but really, we just paid a small fee to get twice as many calories as we need.

Studies have proven that individuals given larger portion sizes will eat more even if they don't particularly like the taste of the food. For example, someone might go to the movies and order a small popcorn. The cashier tells them they should get a large, as it is twice as much, but they only have to pay a dollar more. Not thinking, that customer ends up ordering the largest option of popcorn. Then, during the movie, they realize the popcorn is stale and needs salt. Even though they don't like the way it tastes, that customer still eats the entire large bucket because they don't want to waste their money. This kind of mentality manifests itself in other ways and can be incredibly dangerous for anyone that is trying to diet. We have to be aware of how portion promises and promotions trick us into spending more money.

We also feel a need to finish our plates in order to ensure we're getting our money's worth. We go out to eat and order a plate of pasta, and we decide to get the dinner version. It is way too much, but we still eat the last few bites because it is not enough to justify getting a to-go box, but it is also too much to just dump in the trash. We fear wasting our food (that is going to be wasted anyways), so we eat massive portions just to feel better about saving a few dollars.

When you go out to a restaurant, before you even start eating, split it in half. If you get a burger and some fries, cut it in half and separate the fries. Try to eat only half; that way you can take the other half home. If you halve the portion before you even start eating, you allow yourself to see how much you have left, so you enjoy the bites you take, while still making sure you don't eat too much. Then you will still have more for your money by having an entire second meal at home. By getting into this mental habit, we are better able to track our portions both when going out to eat and when serving ourselves at home.

Even take-home packages are way too large. Always check the portions before eating anything. Just because it is handheld and came from a vending machine does not mean you should be eating it all in one sitting. If you look at the nutrition facts, you might realize that drink you have every morning is actually supposed to be three different servings. We allow our portion perspective to become warped because we use packaged food as a standard.

Some people find success in weight loss by just cutting down portions. That is why certain programs, like Weight Watchers, work so well for many different people. Some people might only eat healthy food, yet they can't figure out what it takes to actually lose weight. Eating only vegetables is still unhealthy if you eat pounds of veggies a day. Your body still takes in everything that you eat, storing, using, and wasting every part of that food. Just because it is healthy does not mean it might not still have some fat that your body chooses to store.

Our brains don't see portions, just plates. If only we had the natural biological urge to perfectly portion out meals like we know that we want to eat, many of us would be a lot better off. Unfortunately, some of our eyes are way bigger than our stomachs, and we don't always know what's best for us in terms of portion control. Many animals have to be monitored about how much food they are given, or else they will eat everything in their bowl until it is empty. This is from a natural instinct to load up on food. Some animals in the wild go days without finding another kill, so they make sure to stuff their bodies so they don't go hungry in between meals. We need to be mindful that part of our brains have this kind of instinct as well. It is not as intense as it is for some animals, but we do still have to be incredibly cautious of the urge to clean our plate.

Eating slow is the best way to make sure that you are not overeating. Let your stomach catch up to your mind. Also, always go with tiny portions. This way, if you want seconds, you can go for it! If you cooked a huge serving of pasta, don't load up your plate. You can always go back and get more! You are also giving yourself the illusion that you are eating more. For example, maybe an average pasta dinner for you is three cups of cooked pasta. Next time you go to eat dinner, start out with just a cup of pasta. Eat slowly, and if you are still hungry, go back for a second round. After that, you will likely not be hungry because the first portion caught up with you. You will also have the idea in your head that you already went for seconds, so you will avoid going up for a third time as it just becomes excessive. You will likely feel full after two cups, even though you have become accustomed to eating three.

Use smaller containers and plates as well. Instead of finding the biggest bowl in your cabinet for your cereal, just use a small cup. If you want a second serving of cereal, you can do so without finishing an entire box in one sitting!

When eating snacks, don't bring the entire container to the couch. Instead, pour your chips into a bowl or cup. If the bag of chips is just sitting next to you on the couch, you are going to eat the whole thing. Instead, if you just fill a cup, when you are done, you will likely just let yourself feel satisfied as you will have to get back up for a second portion.

Chapter 3 – Strategies and Mind Exercises

When we think of weight management, our minds often go to diet and exercise. What's more important than hitting the gym is exercising our brain. If we make sure that the most important organ in our body is taken care of, we can be certain that other healthy habits will soon follow. You can diet, exercise, and do everything else you need to lose weight, but if you continually distract, deflect, or flat out avoid your problems and root issues, you will never find true happiness. The happier you are and the more aware you can be of your mental health, the better it will be in the end which will also lead to an overall better quality of life.

Keep a Journal

Keeping a journey is a healthy habit for many people no matter what their goals, but it's important for someone that wants to lose weight as well. By writing down your different portion measurements and exercise habits, you can better ensure that you'll have a basis for evaluation. When this is done, you can predict future problems that might keep you from your goals by looking back on the days of recorded mistakes or slipups. You can see what kinds of schedules and structures aren't working so you can create better habits in the end. The more extensive your journaling, the better you'll be able to create your own research study of your weight-loss journey, meaning you can share your progress or use it as a structure for future diets.

Avoid the Scale

The biggest issue with weight-loss strugglers comes when they see the number on the scale. Someone that wants to lose ten pounds might get discouraged if they find they only lost nine.

Sometimes, people might even have to gain weight before they end up losing a pound. By avoiding the scale altogether, certain failures and disappointments can be avoided as well.

Find a different way to track your progress. You can have monthly weigh-ins, but it shouldn't be something that should be checked once a day. Our weight fluctuates so much throughout our journey that it isn't worth stressing over on a daily basis. Any checking that happens more than once a day is also likely a bad habit; you're using it to distract yourself from a bigger issue.

The Calorie Myth

When many people diet, they focus too much on calories. They'll see that a certain snack pack only has a hundred calories, which means that it's good for you, right? Wrong. When we focus too much on how many calories are in something, we're failing to look at all the other factors that make up that product. Something with zero calories might include harmful chemicals or hidden substances that are bad for us. Something with a ton of calories might be avoided even though it has a large number of vitamins and necessary fiber.

Calories should still be considered, as the more calories you take in, the more you have to burn through exercise. They still shouldn't be a basis for what foods you decide to eat. If you focus too much on calories, you'll end up losing sight of other important issues. Remember that weight loss isn't about numbers. What's on the scale or on the nutrition package is important in making certain measurements, but they shouldn't be the definitive goals that you're creating on your weight-loss journey.

Talk About It

Keeping things in is never good. In fact, it can feel pretty awful. Those that are overweight might find themselves feeling embarrassed about their weight. Maybe they end up making excuses for themselves when they eat certain foods, verbalizing these reasons to others around them as a form of validation. "Oh, I'll just start my diet tomorrow," you might hear someone say as they sneak a few extra cupcakes from the dessert table. This kind of discussion can be counterintuitive. Instead, try talking about the issues and struggles you have rather than about the way you're going to make up for your problems later. You might find that you end up getting some great advice from a person that's going through a similar struggle.

It's important to be a good listener as well. Sometimes, people aren't looking for answers or advice when they're complaining about their issues. It's nice to just have someone to vent to every once in a while. By creating a discussion, you can more easily tackle the issues that are causing problems in your weight-loss journey.

Avoid telling people about your goal before you get on track, however. Talking about your feelings, emotions, and struggles is always a good thing. Sometimes it just takes saying a thing out loud for it to feel real. However, many people set themselves up for failure by sharing their goals too early. Those that post on social media about how they're going to lose weight are actually less likely to follow through with their goals. Stay silent with the majority in the beginning of your journey, confiding in just those you know you can rely on and trust.

Affirmations

Practicing affirmations is an important mindset strategy in weight loss. An affirmation is a type of positive reinforcement that helps in combating negative thoughts. Instead of telling yourself you're "no good" because you didn't follow through with a small goal, you should give yourself an affirmation such as "I am capable of continuing" to remind yourself of how powerful you really are. Below is a list of positive affirmations you should use in order to combat negative thoughts and improve overall encouragement:

1) I can do this. I am capable of losing weight and I have the ability to reach my goals.
2) I am exercising every day and eating healthy as often as possible. I am actually doing what I should be doing in order to achieve my goals.
3) If I can start my journey, I can finish it.
4) I do not need processed foods to feel happy. I can feel the same joy from cooking a healthy meal.
5) I have exercised before and can do it again. It is hard to start, but I know that once I do, I have what it takes to finish my exercise routine.
6) I am healing myself. I have been through challenging times and deserve to feel happy.
7) I am loved and am full of love.
8) I am losing weight to be healthy.
9) I am beautiful no matter what size. Skipping one day at the gym does not mean that I am not beautiful.
10) I am eating healthy food full of nourishment. I can feel the positive change in my body and I know that I only have more to look forward to.

Chapter 4 – Time Management

The most important part of a weight-loss journey is time management. This doesn't mean setting a quick goal and achieving it as fast as possible. It's all about using time properly and understanding how long it takes to actually do something. We set ridiculous goals for ourselves in the hopes that we'll achieve something great, but what ends up happening is, as the end-date approaches, we become overwhelmed and are set up for disappointment. We have to be realistic with our time goals and consider all factors when making different plans.

Practice Patience

Patience is hard to achieve. Anyone that wants to lose weight hopes that they can just jump on the scale after eating a salad and see the number drop by double digits. We have to accept before starting a weight-loss journey that this will never happen. We won't be able to just lose the weight overnight.

Sometimes, patience is hard to have when exercising. Many people find themselves getting bored on treadmills or other machines that require repetitive activity for minutes at a time. Use different exercise methods that you find fun or entertaining, such as a dance class or going on an interesting trail run. If the gym is your only option, use the boring moments on machines as a way to meditate. Clear your head, not thinking of how much weight you want to lose or what else you have to do to get there. Just practice counting or focusing on a quiet place you find peace in, such as a beach or a park. Visualize this in order to find a place of meditation. It'll take practice, but you'll soon find that you can zone out and work hard if you just focus.

There is No Rush

Weight loss takes time; we can't emphasize that enough. Some diets and exercises will help you lose weight quicker than others, but overall, you're going to have to put in a lot of time to lose weight. Remember not to feel too rushed throughout this journey. You have to be strict and consistent to actually see results, but there's no point in forcing yourself into ridiculous time constraints. If you cause yourself anxiety over certain dates, you might feel the need to stress-eat or go through dangerous dieting practices to get there.

Set Small Goals

Instead of looking at a wedding coming up in a couple of months as your goal for losing weight, instead, use that as a small milestone. Many of us get worried looking at the future, thinking of things coming up as the time limits for which we have to lose weight. Maybe it's March and you only have a couple months until swimsuit season. Instead of going on a diet to lose thirty pounds in three months, use the beginning of summer as a small milestone in your journey. Aim, instead, to be healthier and more confident by the time summer comes, rather than giving yourself a ridiculous goal that you don't even know if you can achieve.

Don't Wait for Monday

Many people have an unhealthy perceptive of dieting when looking at certain periods of time. Maybe it's a Tuesday, and so they tell themselves that next Monday is going to be the date to start dieting. In preparation for that date, that same person might make sure to eat all the junk in their house to make sure temptation is removed. But then, by the time Monday comes, something else happens that delays it further.

Even worse, maybe it's Sunday night and you decide that since tomorrow is Monday, you're going to start your diet right now. But then, Tuesday comes, and the diet doesn't start, so you feel discouraged and you count that as just another time that you failed! Don't do this! Instead, set a starting point much further into the future. Find a date two weeks away, whether it's on a Monday, the first of the month, or just a random Wednesday. That way, you can prepare for the official diet-start date. This way, you can practice as the actual date approaches.

For example, your New Year's resolution might be to lose weight. If that's the case, throughout December, you should practice incorporating workout routines a few times a week and experiment with healthy dinners. Then, when January comes around, you have more experience in dieting and are better prepared to actually start your journey than if you had only given yourself a few days to prep.

Something to Tend

Your weight is something to tend. Think of it like a plant. You don't just plant a flower and walk away. The flower will grow, but if you don't go back and make sure to water it, the flower will die. Your journey is a flower. By purchasing this book, you've purchased the seeds. As you read these words, you're reading how to plant the seed and how to make sure that it stays alive. After you've finished the book, it's time to plant the seed. This is done by creating a workout plan and diet.

Once the flower blossoms, you'll have reached your weight-loss goal. Just like the flower, if you abandon your goals and don't tend to your weight-loss journey, you will fall off track and go back into your old lifestyle.

Lifestyle Change

Losing weight isn't just a reduction in numbers. It's a change in the entire way you live your life. There are some people that seem very thin and yet they might be able to eat whatever they want. These people give the illusion that if an overweight person becomes thin, they can then start to eat what they want. That's not how it works, however. Those thin people are just among the handful of individuals that were just born lucky! If you're overweight now, there's a good chance that it's part of your makeup, and weight fluctuations might just be something you have to learn how to manage.

This means you can't just cut out soda for a year, lose fifty pounds, and then start drinking soda again. The weight will come back if you don't manage your habits. That idea can be scary for some people. They might assume that they have to give up soda forever. That doesn't have to be the case. What has to change is just how much soda you can consume. If you drink a Coke a day, you might want to just give the Coke up, hoping you can go back to that behavior after you lose a certain amount of weight.

You have to accept that you can no longer drink a Coke every day if you want to keep up with your weight. Instead, maybe just have soda on weekends, or only when you're going out to eat. Find a way to incorporate the things you desperately love from your past life into your new healthy lifestyle.

Keeping the Weight Off

The part where many people really fall through with their goals is after they actually achieve them! Many people get to their desired weight, see that number, and think they no longer have to keep up with their diet plan. Then, the weight comes back, and the cycle of disappointment has to be lived all over again. Remember that once you reach your first goal, you should set another one. The second might not be as extreme. For example, maybe your first goal is to get down to 180 pounds. Once you do that, you have to come up with something new. That might be getting down to 170 pounds, or it could be something different, such as improving the muscle mass in a certain part of your body. Never stop setting goals. The level of difficulty can fluctuate. But to stay on track and keep the weight off, you have to continually encourage yourself to do better.

Change Things Up

Some people might find that after a year or two of dieting and exercising, they stop losing weight. This can be because their bodies are now used to the healthy behavior. You probably won't ever lose as much weight in a diet as you do at the beginning. Those transformations can be invigorating, but remember that as you continue, it will become a little less drastic.

If you feel you've plateaued in your diet, you should consider changing things up. This might involve trying an entirely new diet, or it could be working out in a different way. Incorporating variety helps to ensure that you'll stick to your goals while also having fun!

Don't Revel in Regret

Once you reach your weight-loss goals, you might find yourself feeling regretful. Maybe you feel remorse over not doing it sooner. You might think to yourself about how if you had started exercising as a teen, it wouldn't be so hard to keep up with the weight now. Don't blame your past self for what they didn't do. Instead, thank them for what they taught you. There is no going back in time. What happened, the decisions we made, and the weight we gained already occurred, and there's no reversing. Instead, we have to look at our past mistakes and use them as lessons.

Remember that you wouldn't be the person you are right now if you hadn't experienced every single thing you did. The more you learn to love yourself, the better you'll be able to forgive the past "you" for all the things they did you wish they hadn't.

It Gets Easier

Always remember that it will get easier. You just have to get into a healthy lifestyle with good habits. The more practice you put into working out, and the more dedicated you are to your diet, the better you'll be able to manage your weight. The first day at the gym is going to be tough. You might be excited to start, but there also might be feelings of fear of judgment and anxiety that you might fail. Don't let anything discourage you from going back. Each and every time you walk through the doors of your gym or decide *not* to eat the candy in the workroom, remember that next time, it's going to get even easier.

The struggle doesn't end. Your legs will always be sore after an intense workout. You'll still sweat through your T-shirts, and you'll still crave all the sweets that caused the weight gain in the first place. Those difficulties don't just disappear. However, the more dedicated you are and the better focus you have on achieving your goals, the easier it gets each and every time.

<u>Conclusion</u>

While many people think that weight loss is about just working out, the most important key to shed the pounds is in your own brain. Our brains are made up of our experiences, the things we were taught, the things we've seen, and the biology of our brains provided by ancestors and our parents. Our brains are the most important organ in our body. Without then, we are just bodies. Our bodies are also important, but if we don't take care of our brain, we can't truly take care of the rest.

Weight-Loss Mindset Review

There are many different steps to losing weight, but finding the right weight-loss mindset requires a few key steps that are important for everyone, no matter if they're on a ketogenic diet or trying out Weight Watchers. In order to achieve a weight-loss mindset, you must:

1) Look inward. What is it about food that makes it so hard to give up?

2) Figure out the role that food plays in your life. Is it a comfort tool for a past trauma?

3) Evaluate the way you were raised. What triggers have been created that might have led to your current behavior? Look at your parents or the people that raised you. How did their dieting behavior affect you?

4) Be easy on yourself. You're not going to reach your goals by belittling yourself along the way.

5) Practice patience. Accept and understand that it's going to be a struggle. Be kind to yourself if something takes longer than you want it to and be forgiving if you have a slipup. It will take time to reach your goals.

Be Proud of Yourself

No matter where you are in your weight-loss journey, at any given time, you should be proud. Over sixty percent of the U.S. population is overweight, so it's not like you're the only one that struggles to diet and exercise. The fact that you even want to change is something you should be proud of. It's not easy, and if it were, everyone would be thin and healthy. Even though you might want to blame yourself for being here in the first place, remember that positive reinforcement is the way you're going to be able to keep up with your goals.

Remember, it is Up to You

You can use different tools, gym memberships, or workout gear to help encourage you to live a healthier lifestyle. At the end of the day, the only thing you can depend on is yourself. Your motivation, desire, and dedication are the only things that's will help you find the life that you've always wanted, and certainly deserve.

Thank you!

Thank you so much for reading my book!

I hope that you enjoyed the experience. I truly want you to obtain what you need to care for yourself and to regain and/or maintain your health!

Please remember that independent authors live and die (professionally) by the reviews that are left for us.

Please be so kind as to leave a review on Amazon after reading my book.

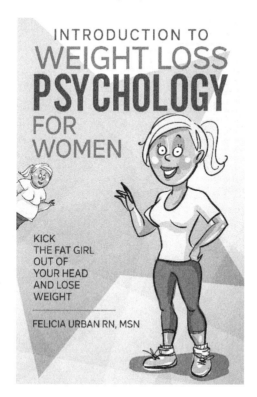

Interested in more content by
Felicia Urban?

Come visit us on the Weight Loss Psychology Series website and don't forget to hit that subscribe button to stay up to date on all new content!

https://WeightLossPsychologySeries.com

Interact with Weight Loss Psychology community by joining the Facebook page

https://www.facebook.com/WeightLossPsychologySeries

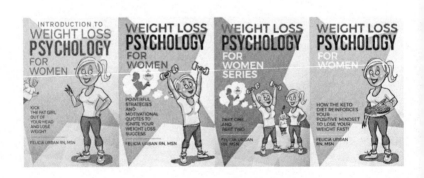

Printed in Great Britain
by Amazon